Herbal Antibiotics & Antivirals

Natural Healing with Herbal Medicine

Christine Weil

Christine Weil

Table of Contents

Introduction

I want to thank you and congratulate you for purchasing, *Herbal Antibiotics & Antivirals: Natural Healing with Herbal Medicine.*

This book contains proven steps and strategies on how to grow, prepare, and dry your medicinal herbs, and how to prepare the various medicinal preparations you can make at home. In addition, this guide will show you how to successfully use these herbs to obtain the most pleasure, benefits and success from all your efforts.

When you fill your life with herbs, they bring beauty to your yard, and yummy flavors to your meals. The medicinal herbs can improve your health, and prevent illness or ease the symptoms when you are ill.

Thanks again for purchasing this book, I hope you enjoy it!

Christine Weil

Understanding Herbal Remedies

Herbs have been studied and used for centuries as medicine and as a food. With the modern use of pharmaceuticals, there was a period of time when herbal medicines was thought of as "old fashioned" and as "quackery".

Within the last few years, herbs have slowly regained popularity and usage. Once again, people are discovering the value of herbal products as a part of their health routine, and as a pleasant craft to study and enjoy.

Herbal remedies use plant parts or the extracts for different health conditions. The most common forms of herbal medicines include poultices, essential oils, creams, tincture, and teas. In the United States, many herbal remedies are sold in stores which sell alternative medications, vitamins, and other similar products.

The medical community in general still disapproves of the use of herbs as medicine. They believe that herbs are ineffective, unsafe, not regulated, and not as effective as pharmaceutical drugs.

The ironic thing about this belief is that many medications prescribed by our physicians have components of herbal remedies or at least a synthesized version of the herb. Before using any herbal remedy, it is wise and recommended that you do some thorough research, and discuss the use of an herb with an herbalist and/or your physician before using. Some herbs can be dangerous if used inappropriately.

Many people consider plant-based remedies to be more natural, cheaper, and less harmful than pharmaceutical drugs. There is also the belief that they are more capable of easing both every day and chronic health problems. Today we have over-used antibiotics to the point where they are losing their effectiveness, and are causing yeast overgrowth in our bodies. Yeast overgrowth can lead to several minor and some serious health conditions. With the use of herbs we don't have to limit ourselves to taking our medicine in a pill.

Herbs boost the natural healing properties of our immune system, so we actually heal faster. The herbs stimulate the necessary healing hormones which fight against the pathogens.

A popular way to administer an herbal remedy is by consuming herbal teas. The leaves or berries of a plant are steeped in hot boiling water for – five to ten minutes. The pot must be covered so that the essential oils don't escape, but rather allows the oils, nutrients, and herbal flavors to be released into the water, which in turn becomes a tea. Many of the herbs used today are sold either as loose leaf teas or in tea bags. When you use loose leaf tea, a steeping ball or straining the loose leaf tea after it has steeped will keep the leaves out of your tea.

Along with lifestyle, dietary, and activity changes, herbs can help to improve our general well-being. These positive changes help us to resist the pathogens which are around us daily.

An herb is a plant with a useful purpose, such as a source of dye, a flavoring to food, a medicine, or an insect repellent. With homegrown herbs, you can prepare a delicious soup, which will be full of flavor, and fill your kitchen with a delightful aroma. They will then fuel the bodies of you and your family with goodness.

Natural Antibiotic Herbs

Believe it or not, you already have an herbal medicine box located at your fingertips. It's in your kitchen! These herbs can help increase your immunity to colds and viruses. Bay leaves are one these medicinal herbs. They have both antibacterial and antifungal properties, and can easily be added to your soups.

Sage is a herb which is popular when used on chicken, turkey, and other poultry. Sage also has antibacterial and antiviral properties. Fresh sage is best, because of the beneficial compounds concentrated in its oils.

As a rule, strongly scented and flavored herbs and spices come with powerful oils which can add flavor, improve your health, and prevent illness. Cinnamon, nutmeg, rosemary, and cloves help boost your immune system. Add some cinnamon, or nutmeg to your oatmeal or hot chocolate, and rosemary to your salad dressing, to help make tasty treats and to add health benefits. Here are some important facts about the best herbs and spices in your spice rack for boosting your immunity, and preventing or treating colds and flu symptoms.

Note: You will notice that many of these herbs are used as a tea, a favored and easy way to consume and receive the health benefits of many medicinal herbs.

Herbal Antibiotics Found in your Spice Rack:

Basil

Basil is highly fragrant plant whose leaves resemble peppermint, a cousin of basil. Basil's rounded leaves are usually green in color, but there are some varieties which have leaves with hints of red or purple. There are 60 varieties of basil. The taste of sweet basil if fresh and pungent. Basil grows in many regions of the world, but is native to India, Asia, and Africa.

Research studies on basil show that that it has unique health-protecting effects in two basic areas - basils *flavonoids* and *volatile oils*. The flavonoids found in basil provide protection at the cellular level. *Orientin* and *vicenin* are two water-soluble flavonoids which have been of particular interest. Research studies of human white blood cells have discovered that basil's flavonoids protect cell structures and chromosomes from radiation and oxygen damage.

Basil has also been shown to provide protection against unwanted bacterial growth. These antibacterial properties are due to the volatile oils which contain estragole, linalool, cineole, eugenol, sabinene, myrcene, and limonene. Lab research has proven the effectiveness of basil in restricting growth of numerous bacteria such as Listeria, E Coli, Pseudomonas, and Staphylococcus,

Essential oil of basil is obtained from its leaves, and has been proven to inhibit several species of pathogenic bacteria now resistant to commonly used antibiotic drugs. Essential oil of basil was even found to inhibit strains of bacteria from the genera enterococcus staphylococcus and pseudomonas, which have shown a high level of resistance to antibiotic drugs

Washing produce in a solution containing just one percent basil essential oil results in dropping the number of Shigell - an infectious bacteria that causes diarrhea.

Including basil in more of your recipes is easy to do and makes good sense. Raw vegetables salads, especially, can benefit from the addition of basil. Adding fresh basil to your salad dressing will also brighten the flavor of your fresh.

Garlic

Garlic gained its famed in Hollywood as a repellant against evil, (imaginary) blood-sucking vampires. In our real world, garlic is most effective in the battle against bacteria and its mutations. These are due to our heavy antibiotic drug use. If we don't stop prescribing antibiotic drugs for every little cough and sneeze, these mutations will grow, multiply, and continue to change until antibiotic drugs are no longer effective against them. Since garlic seems to offer real help with these, let's consider their benefits.

Garlic has been prized for approximately 5,000 years. It is a stimulant for the immune system, and a natural, safe antibiotic. Garlic's strong aroma is mostly due to its sulphur-containing compounds, which account for most of its medicinal properties. Garlic is effective against Tuberculosis, Shigell, Staphylococcus, Pseudomonas, E. coli, Streptococcus, Salmonella, and influenza B.

Garlic is a potent antiseptic. It was used for that purpose in both World War I and World War II. Recent research has revealed that garlic contains vitamin A and C, thiamin and riboflavin.

Garlic may be taken fresh as juice or cloves, in capsules, as tincture or in food. Every garlic preparation's potency depends on the amount of *allicin*, garlic's active ingredient. A milligram of *allicin* is said to be equal to 15 units of penicillin. One clove of fresh garlic daily can be used to control hypertension.

For those who find raw garlic unpleasant, factory-made extracts containing 1.3% of allicin can be used. About 600 milligrams to 1.2 grams of garlic extract may be divided and taken three times a day.

Start with small doses and gradually increase. Garlic is most potent chewed raw. However, raw garlic can cause stomach upset and vomiting if taken in large doses, so start with only ¼ teaspoon raw garlic or juice as needed for antibiotic purposes. Capsules are much easier to tolerate. Cooking with garlic is also an excellent way to add more garlic into your diet and reap its antibiotic benefits.

If you are taking blood thinning medication, consult your physician before adding garlic to your health routine.

Cayenne Pepper

Cayenne pepper is a type of chili pepper plant with red, slim fruits that are used to add flavor to food. This type of pepper is known as the "guinea spice" or the "bird pepper." Its scientific name is *Capsicum anuum*. It is related to paprika and other chilies like the tabasco, bell pepper, and habanero. It is "borderline spicy" at the Scoville scale. Borderline spicy is described as *"extremely hot and dry, even in the fourth degree."*

Cayenne pepper has been used by Native Americans as both a food and a medicine for 9,000 years. The hot and spicy taste of cayenne pepper is due to a substance known as capsaicin, which helps to reduce pain and inflammation.

Capsaicin is the most active ingredient in cayenne. Cayenne also contains vitamins A and C and flavonoids, carotenoids and antioxidant properties.

As a spice, cayenne may be eaten raw or cooked. Dried cayenne pepper is available in powdered form, and can be added to food, stirred into juice, tea, or milk. It is also available in capsule form, and in creams for external use.

Cayenne Pepper Preparations and Dosage

Don't give cayenne to children under two years. Capsaicin ointment may be used on the skin with caution in older children, but don't use capsaicin for more than two days in a row.

Capsaicin cream is useful for adults who are suffering from shingles. One may apply it directly to affected areas up to four times a day. The shingles' pain may be a little intense at first, but it will subside within a few days. It usually takes three to seven days before you notice substantial pain relief and healing.

Have the symptoms of a cold or sinus infection? To clear a head cold and relieve sinus pain and congestion, try drinking a cup of tea made with lemon and either ginger or some horseradish, to which you've added a dash or two of cayenne pepper.

Cold and Flu Tea

2 teaspoons sage leaves, crushed
Juice of one lemon
Pinch cayenne pepper
1 tablespoon honey

To prepare the tea
1. Pour one cup boiling water over sage, cover, and allow to steep for 10 minutes.
2. Strain out the remaining herb.
3. Add remaining ingredients, and drink it while hot.

Cayenne pepper is a time-honored approach to treating disease. It does, however, have some side effects, and can interact with other herbs, supplements or medications. Consult your physician before trying cayenne pepper tea, gargles, capsules, or creams.

Cinnamon

Cinnamon is a pungent and warming herb which is good for all sorts of conditions, from the common cold to stomach upsets.

Cinnamon is also used as an herbal seasoning to spice up sweet and savory dishes. Cinnamon bark, from the *Cinnamomum* tree, tends to curl up as it is dried, making the well-known cinnamon sticks. Cinnamon was first used by the Egyptians around 2000 B.C. Today, Sri Lanka produces approximately 80% of the world's supply of true cinnamon. The cassia variety of cinnamon is mostly grown in Indonesia, and is more popular and more widely used than true cinnamon. Cinnamon bark has been used in folk and alternative medicine as a remedy for treating colds, nausea, and indigestion.

How to use Cinnamon

Adding cinnamon to food is the most common use of this herb. It's delicious in tea, cocoa, desserts, pastry, and in meat dishes. It's a popular spice used extensively in the Mediterranean diet. Cinnamon's flavor and aroma is caused by an essential oil called *cinnamic aldihyde*. This essential oil is a potent antibacterial, antifungal, and uterine stimulant. Inhaling five drops of cinnamon essential oil mixed in boiling water is effective for coughs and respiratory irritation.

To activate your immune system to resist colds, try drinking Cinnamon Tea. It's both warming and delicious.

Cinnamon Tea

½ to 1 teaspoon of cinnamon bark
2 cups of water
Honey to taste

1. Simmer ½ to 1 teaspoon of cinnamon bark in 2 cups of water for 10 minutes.
2. Cover and let steep for 10 minutes.
3. Strain out herb, and pour tea into a cup, add honey to taste, and drink while hot.

1 cup of tea two or three times a day is recommended to resist or treat the symptoms of a cold.

Spiced Cinnamon Apple Tea:

Simple and delicious!

1. Put a quart of brewed tea into a pot.

2. Add 2 cups of apple juice.

3. Gently simmer with a sliced lemon and two cinnamon sticks for 10 minutes.

Enjoy!

Added Benefits of Cinnamon

Researchers conducted a study in 2000 which showed that the extract from cassia cinnamon had a positive effect for the treatment of HIV-1. It continues to be under study. In another study in 2008, cinnamon was shown to have some antiviral effects, and could prevent some strains of fungi, Staphylococci, Clostridium, and Escherichia.

Avoid the use of therapeutic doses of cinnamon essential oil in pregnancy due to its uterine stimulant potential. Use cinnamon with care if you have a high fever.

Ginger

Ginger is originally from Asia, and has been used as a medicinal herb in the West for 2000 years. Ginger was introduced into America by the Spaniards and is now grown in the West Indies. It is a hot, dry herb which was traditionally used to warm the stomach, and relieve chills. In China, the fresh root is used to promote sweating, and as an expectorant for colds.

Ginger is a popular rhizome or tuber to cook with. Whether fresh, dried, or ground, it is used in cuisines around the world. Raw ginger is used in soups, stir-fries, curries, chutney, and in meat and fish dishes. It is loved as a spice in pumpkin pie, with sweet potatoes, and squash. When ginger is dried, it becomes more pungent, making the flavor stronger. This spicy hot ginger is used in Ayurvedic and Chinese medicine for healing.

Benefits of Ginger

Ginger has been used for its warming effect, which in turn, increases perspiration. Healthy sweating, which is often helpful during colds and flus, may do a lot more than simply assist with detoxification. German researchers have recently found that sweat contains a potent germ-fighting agent that may help fight off infections.

Investigators have isolated the gene responsible for the compound and the protein it produces, which they have named *dermicidin*. Dermicidin is produced in the body's sweat glands, released into the sweat, and transported to the skin's surface where it provides protection against invading microorganisms, including bacteria such as *E. coli* and *Staphylococcus aureus*, and fungi, including *Candida albicans*.

Ginger stimulates digestion, respiration, circulation and the nervous system. Many people use ginger tea and candied ginger to reduce inflammation and reduce pain. Ginger is best known for its ability to relieve indigestion, nausea and morning sickness.

As an expectorant, ginger may ease the symptoms of colds, coughs, and the flu. The root acts as an antihistamine and decongestant, two cold-easing effects that can help with symptoms. Ginger is concentrated with active substances. One doesn't have to use very much to receive its beneficial effects.

How to Use Ginger

If possible, choose fresh ginger over the dried form. It is not only better-quality in flavor, but also contains higher levels of *gingerol, the active ingredient in ginger related to capsaicin.* It also has a higher level of *protease,* ginger's active anti-inflammatory compound. Fresh ginger root is sold in the produce section of most supermarkets. When buying fresh ginger root, make sure it is firm, smooth, and free of mold. Ginger is available in two forms, young and mature. Mature ginger, the more widely available type, and has a tough skin that requires peeling. Young ginger, usually only available in Asian markets, does not need to be peeled.

Even through dried herbs and spices like ginger powder are widely available in supermarkets, you may want to explore the local spice stores in your area. Often, these stores feature an expansive selection of dried herbs and spices that are of finer quality and freshness than those offered in regular markets. When purchasing dried ginger powder, try to select organically grown ginger. This will give you more assurance that it has not been irradiated.

Ginger is also available in several other forms including crystallized, candied, and pickled ginger. Fresh ginger can be stored in the refrigerator for up to three weeks if it is left unpeeled. Stored unpeeled in the freezer, it will keep for up to six months.

Dried ginger powder should be kept in a tightly sealed glass container in a cool, dark, and dry place.

Ginger capsules or powder are also available. Do not take ginger with blood thinners without first consulting your health care provider.

Ginger Tea

To make Ginger Tea

1. Peel the skin from a piece of fresh ginger.
2. Cut off a two-inch chunk and slice it into two cups of water.
3. Simmer, covered, for 20 minutes.
4. Remove the slices and pour into a mug.
5. Add honey and a squeeze of lemon to taste.
6. Eat the slices of ginger after drinking the tea.

Drink up to three cups of tea per day, before meals, to relieve the symptoms of a cold, indigestion, or nausea. Enjoy!

Sage

Sage has been used in cooking and in remedies for over 2,000 years in Greece and Italy, and has been considered a cure-all herb.

Sage is a versatile and easy-to-grow herb, versatile in cooking, and a wonder as a medicinal herb. Sage has antibiotic and antiseptic properties and is best known for its decongestant properties in treating colds. Sage is also used for the treatment of sore throat, mouth sores, and canker sores. Sage Honey is a soothing and effective remedy for a sore throat too.

Sage Honey

1 large bunch of fresh sage leaves
Enough honey to cover the leaves

1. Wash and dry the sage leaves, and place them in a small pan with enough honey to cover.
2. Simmer gently for one hour.
3. Allow to cool to a comfortable temperature.
4. Strain the honey into a sterilized jar containing a sprig of sage.

Dosage: Take 1 teaspoon when needed to soothe a sore throat. It is also effective and delicious when used as a sweetener, and as a medicinal in hot lemon drinks when you have a cold or the flu. Take three or four times per day as needed.

Antiviral Herbs

You won't find these herbs in your spice rack, but they can be purchased in many drug stores, health food stores, and some can be grown in your garden.

Some antiviral herbs are still under study and have limited information, while others have been studied for centuries and have been studied extensively. To obtain further information, contact your local credentialed herbalist to discuss the usefulness, dosages, and effectiveness of each herb.

Echinacea

This pretty perennial also known as the Purple Coneflower, was used by the Native Americans for snakebites, fevers, and old, stubborn wounds. Later it was adopted by the early settlers as a medicinal herb used as a home remedy for colds and influenza.

Members of the medical profession in early America relied greatly on Echinacea, but it became less popular with the arrival of pharmaceutical medicine and antibiotics.

Many physicians today are rediscovering the health benefits of Echinacea. It is widely used in alternative medicine as a herbal remedy. In the past 50 years, it has achieved worldwide attention for its antiviral, antifungal, and antibacterial properties. It has been used in AIDS therapy.

Most popular use of Echinacea is for the treatment of infectious diseases, and a weak immune system. Echinacea extractions also are used to help treat influenza, colds, and chronic fatigue syndrome.

Research has shown Echinacea increases and strengthens the body's natural immune system. Echinacea does this by raising the activity of the white blood cells, raising the level of interferon, and stimulating blood cells to surround invading microbes. Echinacea also increases the making of substances the body produces naturally to fight cancers and disease. Researchers found that

Echinacea reduces cold risks by 58%, so if somebody near you has a cold, there is no harm in taking Echinacea as a preventive method for your protection.

Preparations and Dosage

Because Echinacea is not pleasing as a tea, it is most often taken as tincture or as pills. Teas and tinctures, however, appear to be more effective than the powdered herb in capsules. Many herbalists recommend large and frequent doses at the beginning of a cold, flu, sinus infection, bladder infection, or other illness.

For acute cold or flu infection: Take one teaspoon of tincture every one to three hours, or one to two capsules every two to three hours for the first day or two; then reduce the dosage to two teaspoons tincture or six capsules per day.

For a chronic problem: Take ½ teaspoon tincture, or two capsules Echinacea, three times a day for three weeks and then abstain for one week before continuing again.

Side Effects of Echinacea:

Echinacea is considered quite safe, even at high and frequent doses. Some people, particularly those who are allergic to ragweed and list hay fever as a seasonal complaint, may have an allergic reaction to Echinacea -- characteristically, itchy eyes and throat. Regular use of Echinacea may disguise the symptoms of a more serious underlying disease. If you have any recurrent condition, be sure to consult a physician.

Oregano Essential Oil

Oregano essential oil is high in antioxidants, and contains antimicrobial components that fight against colds and coughs. It can also improve digestion issues and can strengthen the immune system and respiratory system.

Researchers have actually referred to it as nature's most powerful antibiotic.

Oregano essential oil's medicinal components include antifungal, antiviral, antibacterial, anti-inflammatory, and antiseptic. It's also an immune system stimulant.

Oregano oil is helpful in fighting against viruses in which an antibiotic is ineffective. Oregano oil is effective in treating strep, pneumonia, staph and MRSA - which is resistant to many pharmaceutical antibiotics. Oregano essential oil has powerful infection fighting properties for the treatment of colds, bacterial and viral pneumonia, bronchitis, and even athlete's foot.

When Oregano essential oil is used aromatically, it can help decrease airborne pathogens and boost your immunity. Oregano essential oil blends well with Basil, Fennel, Lemongrass, Rosemary and Thyme essential oils.

If you have a cough, here is an effective remedy: Put one drop of Oregano essential oil into a teaspoon of honey or a small glass of water and swallow. For a sore throat place one drop of Oregano essential oil in two ounces of water and gargle.

Have you ever heard of the Flu Bomb?

The Flu Bomb can knock out case of the flu before it becomes severe.

To Make The Flu bomb:

Combine in an empty gelatin capsule

3 drops of Oregano oil
5 drops of On Guard oil
5 drops of Melaleuca (or Tea Tree) oil
5 drops of Lemon oil

Take this concoction every hour at the beginning of the flu symptoms and then every three to four hours until the remaining symptoms are gone, and you are feeling better.

Note: The essential oils and empty gelatin capsules are all available for purchase in health food stores or online herbal stores. Use with caution and read the label directions before use.

Goldenseal

Goldenseal is also known as yellowroot, cycbalm, goldenroot, Indian turmeric, ground raspberry, and orangeroot. Goldenseal is a perennial herb originating in the wooded areas of the Ohio River Valley and other locations in the northeastern United States.

Goldenseal was used by American Indians medicinally as a diuretic, a stimulant, and a wash for sore or inflamed eyes as early as 1793. The Cherokees used goldenseal to cure snakebites, while the Iroquois used it to treat diarrhea, fevers, and pneumonia. Goldenseal was also used to heal arrow wounds and ulcers.

Indians also used the yellow dye produced by the plant. Early settlers learned about the root, and later it found its way into the 19th century pharmacies. In the 19th century, goldenseal was used for gonorrhea and urinary tract infections.

Goldenseal has been used in cold and flu preparations because of its ability to suppress mucus.

Goldenseal is now one of the top selling herbs in the United States for a wide variety of uses. Goldenseal mouthwashes and sterile eyewashes are available over the counter for the treatment of disorders involving the mucus membranes of the eyes, mouth, ears, nose and throat.

Recommended dosages vary from 250 to 1000 mg three times daily. For the flu, 10 to 30 drops of the extract two to four times a day has been recommended.

Adverse reactions to goldenseal are uncommon, yet at very high doses goldenseal may cause nausea, anxiety, seizure or paralysis. Goldenseal is not recommended for women who are pregnant or nursing.

How does it work?

It is believed that Goldenseal's major healing properties are alkaloid compounds called hydrastine and berberine. Researches studies showed that Goldenseal can kill microbes, reduce inflammation, and stimulate the immune system. The alkaloids are quite astringent, and help reduce inflammation of the mucus membranes.

Goldenseal is a potent plant, and must be used with care. Eating the fresh plant can cause inflammation of the mucous membranes. The most common and the safest way to take goldenseal by capsule form. As with many herbal medications, don't exceed three weeks of continuous use without a break of at least two weeks.

Eucalyptus

Eucalyptus is a native of Australia and has been used by Aborigines as a remedy for colds, sore throats, coughs, and bronchitis. Eucalyptus is rich in a volatile oil known as eucalyptol. The world's main source of eucalyptus oil comes from the tree *Eucalyptus globulus.* For centuries the leaves of the eucalyptus were made into a tea claimed to reduce fevers.

Eucalyptus oil should be an important part of your herbal home remedy arsenal, due to its antibiotic, antifungal, antiseptic, antiviral, and antibacterial properties. Eucalyptus works well when used as a decongestant and expectorant to ease coughs and cold symptoms. Its effects in the upper respiratory system have made it indispensable for conditions such as Whooping Cough, Asthma, and Tuberculosis.

The oils of Eucalyptus should never be taken or used without diluting it.

PURE EUCALYPTUS OIL IS DANGEROUS AND AS LITTLE AS 3.5 MILLILITERS CAN CAUSE DEATH. FOR CHILDREN, ESPECIALLY, INGESTING

EUCALYPTUS IS UNSAFE AND SHOULD NOT BE GIVEN TO CHILDREN.

For adults, diluted eucalyptus can be ingested for as long as three months without causing harm.

Eucalyptus oil applied near the throat or the nostrils allow the essential oils to be inhaled, which helps relieve an inflamed respiratory system. Approximately five drops of the essential oil is recognized as a therapeutic dose. Here in the United States it has become a widely-used ingredient in lozenges, syrups, rubs, and vapor baths to relieve the symptoms of a cold or the flu.

Fresh leaves in teas and gargle have been prescribed by herbalists to relieve sore throats, sinusitis, and bronchitis. Adults using eucalyptus oil may dissolve 15 to 30 drops to half of a cup of sesame, almond, or olive oil before it can be used on the skin.

PURE EUCALYPTUS OIL WILL BURN THE SKIN.

Studies on Eucalyptus

The major properties of eucalyptus are eucalyptol, pinene, limonene, citronellal, cryptine, and piperitone. The aroma of eucalyptus oil is similar to camphor.
Researchers have discovered that the eucalyptol from the essential oils have the ability to break up viscous phlegm. Asthma sufferers who have used eucalyptol have been able to lower their use of corticosteroids, with the approval of their physician.

Ways to use Eucalyptus

Eucalyptus is cooling, and inhaling the vapors from a few drops of the essential oil helps to break up the mucus, ease headaches, and the pressure and pain from sinusitis.

To use as a decongestant: pour freshly boiled water over a handful of crushed eucalyptus leaves in a large bowl; cool slightly then place a towel over your head and the bowl, and breathe deeply.

Eucalyptus oil can be used to replace antibacterial cleaners, which are hard on your health.

To use Eucalyptus oil for cleaning:

2 cups water
¼ cup liquid castile soap
1 tablespoon tea tree essential oil
10 drops Eucalyptus oil

Combine the ingredients in a plastic spray bottle and shake well. Spray on the surface and wipe it clean with a damp cloth or sponge.

Licorice Root

Licorice root is an often forgotten medicinal herb today. Greek, Egyptians, Chinese, and other Asian cultures have been using Licorice root for medicinal purposes for centuries. Licorice root contains many compounds such as flavonoids, essential oils, plant sterols, glycyrrhizic acid, and glycosides. The most common use of licorice is to treat coughs, cold, and the flu. This licorice is not the same as the sugary candy confection which is actually flavored with anise.

Researchers suggest that saponin glycosides in Licorice root have expectorant properties which may help with coughs, bronchitis, and asthma. Licorice is known for its antiviral, antibacterial, anti-inflammatory, antispasmodic, antioxidant, and expectorant activity. Preliminary studies have shown that

Licorice root may suppress the multiplication of HIV, and may be beneficial for people with AIDS.

A simple remedy for respiratory infections, sore throat, cold, and flu-type ailments is Licorice Root tea. You can make this tea simply by pouring boiling water over the licorice root. To obtain greater benefits however simmer the Licorice root and its bark for 10 minutes, or try the delicious tea below.

Licorice Root Tea

1 cup of chopped dry licorice root
½ cup cinnamon chips
½ cup dried orange peel
2 tablespoons whole cloves
½ cup chamomile flowers

1. Mix everything together in a bowl.
2. Store in a glass jar, away from light and heat.

To prepare tea:

1. Combine 3 heaping tablespoons of the tea mix and two to five cups of cold water in a saucepan.
2. Bring to a boil over medium heat.
3. Reduce heat to low, and simmer for 10 minutes.

4. Pour into a large cup through a strainer.
5. Sweeten as desired.
6. Drink a cup two to three times per day while ill.

Tea Tree Essential Oil

Tea trees were used for centuries as Australian Aboriginal remedies. They have had a medicinal reputation since the earliest days of European involvement with Australia. The primary active component of tea tree oil is a terpene. This has a strong antiseptic action. The monoterpene p-cymene which makes up a small part of the essential oil also has powerful antibacterial effects. Tea tree oil appears to have both antiviral and antifungal agents, and is well tolerated on the skin.

Tea tree oil is useful for the treatment of infections and inflammation of the skin, and of the respiratory tract and mouth. Tea tree oil made into a lotion or cream has antifungal properties, and is effective when used topically for the treatment of athlete's foot or nail infections.

Tea tree oil can be used as a mouthwash for oral thrush.

1. Dilute three drops tea tree oil in ½ cup warm water.
2. Swish around your mouth for 60 seconds.
3. Spit out. Do not swallow.
4. Repeat four times daily.

Warning: Do not ever swallow tea tree oil.

Chamomile

Stress can actually weaken the immune system. This natural, tasty relaxant could be your answer for the relief from stress.

Known more as a pleasant-tasting tea than as a medicine, chamomile can be effective as a cream for inflamed skin, wounds, and irritation.

Many Europeans and Americans enjoy this apple-scented chamomile tea which is made from the dried or fresh chamomile flowers. People have used chamomile for centuries as a gentle sleep aid as well as to ease indigestion, promote urination, and relieve colic.

When chamomile is used as a tea, it acts as a mild sedative, which helps to ease the anxiety and nervous stress which interferes with your normal sleep pattern.

Chamomile is easy to grow in your herb garden. Making a tea from the flowers picked from your garden is easy to do. Pour one cup of boiling water over one heaping teaspoon of dried chamomile flowers, steep, covered, for 10 minutes, then strain into a cup. Sip this tea three to four times a day to relieve an upset stomach, or drink a cup one hour before going to bed to relax.

Don't use Chamomile if you have an allergy to the pollen of the aster family members such as ragweed.

Chamomile tea:

1. Take one bag, or one to two teaspoons of dried flowers
2. Add 1 cup of boiling water.
3. Steep a few minutes and drink (may be taken as often as you desire).

Calendula

Calendula was named by the Romans in honor of the plant's ability to bloom on the first day of every month.

Calendula can be used as a first aid for wounds, to prevent infection, and to treat pink eye. Calendula can be prepared a few different ways, which include infusions, tinctures, lotions, and ointments. There are no known precautions when using Calendula as a medicinal herb.

Calendula petals do not have a very strong flavor or fragrance. They are commonly used in salads to add color more than to add flavor. It is also delicious with green vegetables. The dried petals can be added to rice to add coloring.

Calendula tea: Steep one to two teaspoons of dried flowers in one to two cups of hot water for 10 minutes. Drink as needed.

Cat's Claw

Cat's claw has antibacterial, antifungal and antiviral qualities in addition to known properties which can boost the immune system increasing your body's protection against illness.

Cat's claw is usually taken internally as a tea, tincture, or a capsule.

Don't use cat's claw while pregnant.

Lemon balm

Lemon balm has been used as far back as the middle ages to relieve stress, anxiety and ease indigestion, due to its calming properties. Lemon balm is a favorite of bee's everywhere, and has been popular with herbalists for thousands of years. It was believed to enhance longevity; a Swiss physician of the early 1500's made an elixir to make man immortal or at least almost immortal as he thought. Lemon balm is native to the Mediterranean region, western Asia, southwest Siberia and northern Africa. Today it is also widely grown in North America and has gained popularity here.

It is a utility herb, useful for so many purposes. Lemon balm is a member of the mint family, so it has the potential to take over your herb garden.

Fresh lemon balm is the best-tasting and most effective form of the medicinal.

Dried lemon balm is of use, but after it is dried, it loses its delicious aroma.

Lemon balm has an important essential oil which contains antiviral components.

Lemon balm has been used to reduce fevers and treat colds, and is effective when treating cold sores. Studies have shown that an ointment made of lemon balm is effective in treating herpes simplex. Lemon balm has proven to be one of the safest herbs, with no known side effects of toxic symptoms. Consult your herbalist or physician before taking if you are pregnant.

Lemon balm makes a yummy tea which can relieve an upset stomach and promote calming. Fresh lemon balm can be used in tinctures, distillates, vinegars and syrups.

Lemon Balm Tea: Pour a cup of boiling water over a small handful of fresh lemon balm leaves or 1 to 2 teaspoons of dried leaves and steep covered for 10 minutes. This tea is delicious iced or hot, sweetened as desired.

Cranberry

Cranberry is a sour fruit grown in wet meadows in North America.

Cranberry has been used for centuries as a potent defense against urinary tract infections due to its ability to make the bladder lining slippery, so that bacteria won't stick to the bladder lining. Cranberry is full of antioxidants and antiviral properties, plus it prevents plaque formation on your teeth. Cranberry can be taken internally by a capsule or by unsweetened juice form.

Elderberry

Elderberry flowers have been used as cordials and teas for centuries, but the tiny black elderberries are less commonly used. The berries contain many of the same essential properties as the flowers, and have been used as anti-inflammatory for sore throats, to soothe coughs, and for bronchial infections and to loosen sinus congestion.

Elderberry is used as a powerful remedy for viral infections like the flu and cold and has been known to shorten the onset of the flu. Elder stimulates the circulation, and causing sweating, which cleanses the body.

Elderberry syrup is the common method for taking Elderberry as a medicinal. The recommended dosage is one to three tablespoons taken per day during the infection.

Elderberry is extremely useful for children and the elderly, especially during the winter months. Take as tinctures or for children make it into syrup.

Caution: Unripe berries may cause vomiting and diarrhea.

Elderberry Throat Gel:

1. Fill a small Mason jar with **ripe** elderberries.
2. Cover with diluted gelatin.
3. Leave in a warm place for two weeks.
4. Pour into a sterilized bottle.

Adults: Take 2 teaspoons three times per day for coughs and sore throats.

Yarrow

Yarrow is a member of the aster family. Many people consider yarrow a perennial weed because it grows wild in fields, alongside the road, in ditches, and meadows.

Yarrow's generic name *Achillea millefolium* comes from the legend that Achilles used a poultice of the plant to stop the bleeding of his soldiers' wounds during the Trojan War. Researchers have discovered that an alkaloid called achilleine in

Yarrow is responsible for stopping the bleeding.
It has been found that Yarrow contains more than 120
chemical compounds proven to reduce inflammation, muscle
spasms, and relieve pain.

Yarrow also can reduce the symptoms of a cold or the flu
when it's consumed as a hot tea. It brings down temperature,
encourages sweating and eases congestion.

The essential oil of Yarrow can be made into a chest rub for
bronchial complaints and coughs.

Yarrow is available as an essential oil or as capsules from
natural food stores.

Caution: Don't use Yarrow during pregnancy.

Growing Herbs

Early settlers brought herbs to America to use as remedies for illness, as dyes, covering for their floors, to preserve and flavoring foods and to add aromas to their homes. Herbal gardens were an important part of each pioneer home. The herb gardens were placed close to their homes in a sunny area for easy access.

As our modern world advanced, an interest in gardening waned, due to the advent of supermarkets and grocery stores, stocked with all the herbs and spices one needs for their kitchen. Dried and fresh herbs were easy and inexpensive to buy without the extra work involved in garden. Today, gardening is gaining popularity. People are finding that gardening is fun, an excellent exercise, and a rewarding endeavor.

Before launching into an elaborate production of growing herbal plants, you need to make a plan. Take stock of your backyard, patio, terrace, balcony window box, or even you kitchen windowsill, before you buy the seeds or plants.

The advantages of growing your own medicinal herbs will be the time and money you can save by stocking your backyard or windowsill with the basic healing herbs. These herbs can treat common ailments such as colds, the flu, inflammation, pain, and infections. Growing herbs may seem difficult, preparing the teas or tinctures may seem complex and confusing, but the truth is you don't have to be a chemist to grow, harvest, and use herbs for medicinal purposes.

Yet growing herbs for medicinal use doesn't have to be difficult. It can be as simple as buying a herbal start, planting it in a window box or windowsill pot, and then taking off small snips of the herb as it grows, to use as a tea.

Herbs for Beginning Gardeners

Beginning herb gardeners may have a difficulty deciding which herbs to plant because of the large quantity of herbs from which to decide on. If you don't have a large area for a garden, you can tuck herbal plants where ever you have soil, sun and access to water. Many of these plants do well in containers. One way to start an herbal garden is by shopping are your local nursery and purchase seedlings. Buy one or two to start, and increase as you begin to feel more confident with the growing process.

It is best to plant herbs in the spring because many are cool weather plants. Hot weather can make these herbs bolt (turn to seed), before you are ready to harvest them. Cool season herbs are include dill, chervil, and coriander. Warm weather herbs include basil and fennel. Talk with the nursery person to find out which herbs grow best in your area, before you buy.

Before you plant the seeds or seedlings, prepare the soil in a weed free, smooth seed bed of crumbly soil, enriched with organic matter and fertilizer. Growing organic ensures that you won't serve friends, family, or yourself pesticide tea. Mark your rows with a string line, as you would if you were planting vegetables. Using a hoe, dig a shallow depression in the soil along the string line. Sow the seeds or plant the seedlings in the bottom of the depression. Lightly cover the seeds or seedlings with soil and gently tamp the soil with the flat part of the hoe. Label the rows with the name of the herb, and the date it was planted. Gently water the area, and keep it moist until the seedlings appear. If you planted seeds, then thin the plants when they are one to two inches tall, spacing them four inches apart.

Herbs do well if not over watered. A plant with shallow roots will need more water than one with a deep root system. When the weather is hot, or there are brisk winds, the soil dries quickly. These are the times to increase the amount of water you apply. The best time to water your plants is in the morning, as watering at night can lead to fungus growth or plant rot.

Check frequently for weed growth and remove them when they are young and small. Staying on top of weeding will help your garden to stay healthy.

Cutting and Division

The cutting and the division of fast multiplying herbs is useful when propagating certain herbs. When seeds are slow to develop, cuttings may be the answer. On the other hand, some herbs multiply rapidly enough to make dividing up a main source of propagation. Propagation also makes it easier to share plants with friends and family. Tarragon, chives, and mint should be divided while lavender should be cut.

Winter Protection

Perennial and biennial herbs should be winter protected. Many herbs are shallow-rooted, which makes them at risk to crowding during spring thaws. Mulch the garden with straw, oak leaves, or evergreen boughs approximately four inches deep to protect the plants. Apply the mulch after the ground has frozen in early winter. Do not remove the mulch until plants show signs of growth in early spring. Early removal could result in some early frost damage.

Growing Herbs Indoors

Herbs can also be grown indoors for year-round enjoyment. Growing herbs indoors is no more difficult than growing them in the garden. Indoor plants will need basically the same environment as herbs grown outdoors; sunlight and a well-drained soil mix that is not too rich.

Select a south or west window. Different herbs have different light requirements, but most need a sunny location. In winter, "grow lamps" or fluorescent lamps are helpful in supplying the light. Herb plants need sun during the summer months. To prevent the loss of foliage and avoid plant damage, bring herbs indoors before frost. A light frost is helpful on mint, chives, and tarragon, as it tends to induce a rest period, and make the resulting new growth firm and fresh.

When planting, mix two parts potting soil and one part coarse sand. There should be an inch of gravel at the bottom of each pot to ensure good drainage. Consider the water needs of each herb. Growing plants need more water as do plants in clay pots or hanging baskets. Misting and grouping the plants on a tray of moistened pebbles will help keep them in a humid condition. Don't over-water your herb plants as it can cause the roots to rot.

You can maintain an indoor herb garden indefinitely by periodic light feeding, yearly repotting, renewing annuals, seasonal moves outdoors for perennials, and occasional pruning. Water plants as needed. Use several planters or a divided one to allow for different moisture needs of plants.

Once your herb garden or windowsill garden gets growing, you can harvest from it almost every day if you desire.

Key points to consider before you decide to use or grow your own herbs:

1. Know your herbs. Before planting herbs in your garden, educate yourself. Know how herbs grow, the conditions for ideal growth, and how to use the herb once you harvest it. With education you learn how to safely use herbs.

2. Provide the right conditions. Herbs grow best when the light, soil, drainage, and climatic conditions meet the herbs requirements for healthy growth.

3. Provide the proper care. Watering, pruning, pinching, harvesting, and providing winter protection for your herbs can help ensure healthy vigorous plants year around.

4. Experiment in the kitchen. Herbs used for cooking, baking and flavoring shouldn't be intimidating. Start with small portions of herbs and spices until you feel sure of yourself and enjoy their flavor. Some herbs with be sweet, bitter, hot, or tart. Learn which flavors are pleasant to your family's palate and your own.

5. For healing, use the right herb in a proper, safe manner. Herbs can be potent or mild. To avoid problems and to successfully treat a condition, use only the herbs suggested for each ailment at the recommended doses.

6. Use herbs throughout your home. Besides being useful in your kitchen and medicine cabinet, herbs often have pleasant fragrances and wonderful beauty.

7. Enjoy the beauty of herbs growing in your garden. Taking a walk around your garden area can be

relaxing and pleasant for your senses. Herbs can regenerate your spirit and life.

Harvesting and Preserving Herbs

Harvesting Herbs

The best time to harvest herbs is when you need them, fresh herbs have the fullest flavors and fragrances when the leaves are young. Fresh leaves may be picked as soon as the plant has enough foliage to maintain growth. If you have an outdoor herb garden, to ensure good oil content, pick leaves or seeds after dew has disappeared, but before the sun becomes too hot. The herbs' essential oils are strongest when the plants are cool. That's why the best time to pick them is in the morning.

In a mild climate, evergreen herbs such as rosemary and thyme can be gathered fresh all year. In colder climates, unless they are grown indoors, they must be harvested before the winter. The leaves of most perennial herbs can be picked at any time during the growing season, and you can cut as much as ¾ of the plants current growth. For leaves such as basil, thyme, sage, mint, and lemon balm, the peak time to pick the leaves is before they flower.

For medicinal purposes use, gather the whole plant before it begins flowering. Gather roots such as licorice in the Autumn as the top growth dies. Gather seeds on a dry day after the seed head colors have changed from green to brown or gray. Cut the stalks before the seeds begin to fall off. Tie the stalks in small bunches, hang upside down, and tie a paper bag over the seed head to collect the seeds as they fall from the heads. Always wash dirty leaves and seed heads in *cold* water, and drain thoroughly before drying.

Preserving the Herbs

Freezing

For preserving tender leaves such as those on fennel, dill, basil, and chives, freezing is the best method to use to preserve their flavor and essential oils. Chop the herbs on a small tray, freeze, then shake the frozen leaves into a resealable plastic bag. When needed, the frozen herbs will be ready for use without the need to thaw them or chop them. Another handy method is, once you chop up the herbs, place them into the compartments of an ice tray and fill them with water, and then freeze.

Drying

The drying of herbs works well for most herbs, except for the tender leaf herbs. Herbs need to be dried in a warm, dry, dark place with good ventilation. For long stemmed and bushy herbs such as sage, rosemary, thyme, the mints, and summery savory, make small bunches, and tie them with a string. Hang the herbal bunches upside down.

With soft-stemmed herbs such as chamomile, lay them out on a wire cooling rack or a drying tray which will allow the air to circulate around the herbs. Dry the herbs away from the direct sun, in a shaded area. The leaves are ready when they are dry and brittle, and the flowers should rustle like tissue paper. Most herbs take about four or five days to dry. Herbs with thicker leaves may take as long as a week or two.

Hang the herbs with seed heads in paper bags in a dry, airy place until they are thoroughly dry and the seeds are falling off their heads or pods. If your area is humid, it is best to dry the herb quickly, using a cool oven or food dehydrator at a temperature of 90 degrees, for one to three days, turning once or twice daily.

Roots need to be wiped or washed clean, then cut lengthwise, and sliced into small pieces. Lay the pieces of root on drying trays, and dry in the oven or food dehydrator set at 130 degree. Stir the pieces every couple of hours until they have lost their elasticity and snap rather than bend between the fingers. You can tie roots in bunches to dry, but it will take much longer.

Storage

When completely dry, the leaves may be screened to a powder, or stored whole in airtight containers, such as canning jars with tightly sealed lids.

Seeds should be stored whole, and ground as needed. Leaves retain their oil and flavor if stored whole, and crushed just before use.

For a few days, it is very important to examine daily the jars in which you have stored dried herbs. If you see any moisture in the jars, remove the herbs and repeat the drying process. Herbs will mold quickly in closed jars if not completely dry.

Once you are sure the herbs are completely dry, place them in the airtight containers, and store them in a cool, dry place away from light. Never use paper or cardboard containers for storage, as they will absorb the herbs' aromatic oils

Herbal Preparations

Although many herbs and spices are safe to use, care is needed. The herbal preparations which are discussed in this chapter are for minor ailments or for prevention of illness, in small amounts. These preparations can be safely used at home, using herbs you can grow yourself with, and methods that are simple and safe to use.

Infusions:

The most common form of herbal preparation, an infusion, is a tea made from fresh or dried leaves, flowers, or soft stems of herbs. Infusions can be used internally or externally for a wide range of conditions.

To make an infusion
1. Warm a teapot with hot water
2. Drain
3. Add 1 ounce dried or 3 ounces fresh herbs.
4. Pour in 2 ¼ cups water that has just begun to boil.
5. Cover and infuse for 10 minutes.
6. Strain.

Take up to three six-ounce cups daily, hot or cold, sweetened with honey or sugar if desired.

Store unused infusion in the refrigerator for up to two days.

Steeping with the teapot covered prevents the herb's essential oil, the medicinally active component, from evaporating. If you can smell the aroma of the herb while it is steeping, you know that some of its essential oils are escaping.

Decoctions:

Decoctions are different from infusions in that the water containing the herb is boiled. This method is used for tougher plant materials such as roots, barks, and berries which require a robust extraction. The high heat increases the extraction of most of the medically useful substances, but it drives off more of the essential oils than in the preparation of an infusion. Decoctions are not suitable for tender herbs such as mints, or lemon balm, because the essential oils are an important component of these herbs.

To make a decoction
1. Place 1½ ounce of fresh or ¾ ounce of dried herbs in a saucepan with 3 cups of cold water.
2. To extract as much of the active components as possible, use chopped or cut herbs.
3. Bring to a boil, and simmer for 20 to 30 minutes, or until the decoction is reduced by a third (about 2 cups).
4. Strain off the liquid, and discard the herb.

The decoction will keep in a clean covered bottle in a refrigerator for two to three days.

Dosage: Take up to three 6-ounce cups daily, hot or cold, with sweetener if desired.

Syrups:

Syrups are a double-strength infusion or decoction of fresh or dried herbs, sweetened with honey or sugar, then cooked to a syrupy consistency. Syrups are soothing to the throat and more palatable. It's also a method which keeps herbs longer, due to the sweetener which act as a preservative.

To make syrups
1. Gently heat 2 cups of an herbal infusion or decoction with 1 and 1/3 cups of honey, or 2 cups of unrefined sugar,
2. Stir until the honey or sugar has dissolved
3. Cool and then strain into a sterilized dark glass bottle or jar sealed with cork stoppers.

Don't use screw tops. If the syrup ferments, and the bottle or jar is covered with a screw top, it could explode from the pressure build-up of the fermentation.

Tinctures:

A tincture is a solution made by steeping any part of an herb in a mixture of alcohol and water. It can be used internally or externally for a wide range of conditions. Tinctures are handy because they are concentrated, so only small amounts are needed. The alcohol dissolves the essential oils from the herb, and since no heat is used, less of the essential components are lost. Since the alcohol acts as a preservative, tinctures can be stored in a dark sealed bottle for up to two years.

Tinctures are made by letting the herb soak in alcohol for a period of time to extract the active ingredient.
To make a standard tincture

1. Cover 10 ounces of fresh herbs, or 5 ounces of dried herbs with 1 quart (1 liter) of 70 to 80 proof alcohol (*Vodka is ideal because of all the spirits it has the least flavor.*

If the herbs are bitter, you may mask the flavor of the herb by using rum or brandy.)

2. Store the mixture in a sealed container for two weeks
3. Then strain through a muslin bag and squeeze out the liquid.
4. Discard the herb
5. Pour the tincture into a sterilized, dark glass bottle for storage in a cool dark place.

Dosage: Take 1 teaspoon two to three times a day, preferably diluted in a glass of water or fruit juice. Tinctures contain only a relatively small of alcohol.

Poultices:

A poultice is a warm, moist quantity of herbs applied directly to an affected area of the body and held in place with a cloth. Suitable herbs are those used for skin problems and for aches and pains.

To make a poultice you don't need exact measurements.
1. Just take a quantity of fresh or dry herbs that will cover the affected area in a thick layer.
2. Place these in a saucepan, add just enough boiling water to cover the herbs, and simmer for two to three minutes.
3. Allow the herbs to cool slightly, squeeze out the excess water, and place the warm cloth firmly around the herbs to hold them in place.

Application: Apply to the affected area every few hours as needed.

Ointments:

An ointment is a soft, oily, or fatty mixture which contains the dissolved components of some healing material. An ointment contains the extraction of fresh or dried herbs in white petroleum jelly, used externally for bruises or skin conditions. Ointments do not contain water so they provide a protective layer on the skin it is applied to.

Herbs used often in ointments are chamomile, calendula, and St John's Wort.

To make an ointment

1. In a double boiler or a glass bowl set over a pan of boiling water, melt 1 ounce of beeswax and 1 cup of olive oil together

2. Add 5 ounces of fresh chopped herbs or 2½ ounces of chopped dried herbs. Gently heat for a couple of hours, stirring frequently

3. Remove from heat, and strain the mixture through muslin into a jar.

4. Quickly pour the ointment into sterilized screw top jars.

5. Wait to tighten the lids until the ointment is cooled.

The ointment will keep up to three months if stored in a cool dark place in dark glass jars or in a dark location.

Application: Apply to affected area two or three times a day.

Washes and Compresses:

Washes and compresses are strained herbal infusions or decoctions which are used for localized pain relief, and are soothing when applied to an affected body part.

Soak a clean piece of soft cotton fabric in the herbal liquid.

Squeeze out the excess, fold into a pad, and place on the area, repeating until relief is felt.

They are especially effective when they are cold, so re-soak the cloth frequently to keep it cool, and reapply as needed.

Creams:

Creams are emulsions of water and oil or fat that like ointments contained the dissolved components of an herbal substance. Creams do not have a water resistant layer effect, instead they partly absorb into the skin, letting the skin breathe and sweat.

To make a cream

1. In a double boiler or a glass bowl set over a pan of boiling water, melt 5 ounces of emulsifying wax, 2 ½ ounces of glycerin, and 5 tablespoons of water together
2. Add 3 ounces of chopped fresh herbs or 1 ½ ounces of dried herbs
3. Heat gently for two hours, stirring frequently
4. Remove from the heat
5. Strain the mixture through muslin into a bowl.
6. Stir the strained mixture slowly until it is cold.

7. If the mixture become too thick work in more water until the consistency is thick and creamy.
8. Place the cream into sterilized screw-top jars (preferably in dark glass jars) using a narrow knife or spatula.
9. The cream will keep up to three months if stored in a refrigerator.

Application: Apply to the affected area two to three times per day.

Weighing the Ingredients:

You may be wondering why the ingredients are measured by weight rather than by volume. Measuring herbs in the form of teaspoons, tablespoons, and cups wouldn't be accurate measurements. One ounce of a dry herb is quite different in volume from an ounce of dried whole leaves or bulky flowering tops.

Dried herbs are more concentrated than fresh herbs, so you must make sure whether the amounts called for in a herbal preparation are dried or fresh.
Usually you will use twice as much fresh herb as you would dry herbs. An ounce of most dried herbs would equal two handfuls of the herb. Why? Dried herbs weigh very little. For the infusions and decoctions you would use much more than you would if you were making an herbal tea.

Conclusion

Thank you again for purchasing this book!

I hope I was able to help you to understand the wonderful benefits of using herbs for medicinal purposes. There is much more that we need to learn about herbal antibiotics, so keep reading and discovering more about the expanding whole of herbal medicine.

Herbs can be effective remedies, especially if it is an infection which doesn't improve through the use of standard treatments and medications. Planting, growing, harvesting, storing and preparing the herbal preparations are all valuable learning experiences for anyone who wants to take charge of their health.

As always, take caution when using herbs as medicine, and be extra careful when using herbal medicine if you are on prescription medication.

If you learn all you can about herbal antibiotics and antiviral herbs, you won't find yourself a victim as more and more drugs become ineffective due to our over usage in our society. Instead you will be able to fill that void with the use of medicinal herbs, because you sought out this education.

The next step is to discover more of the exciting and inspiring books on Amazon about herbs and their purpose in our lives.

Finally, if you enjoyed this book, please take the time to share your thoughts and post a review on Amazon. It'd be greatly appreciated!

Thank you and good luck!

Christine Weil

Check out the other books in the Natural Health & Natural Cures Series

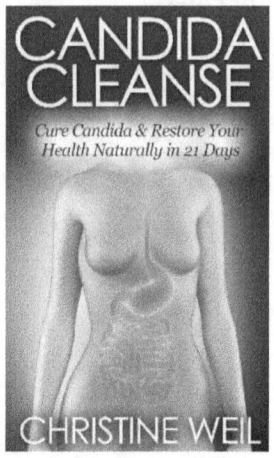

http://www.amazon.com/dp/B00IIRQH9K

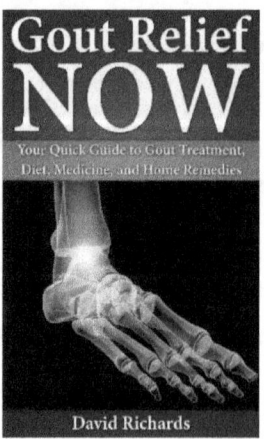

http://www.amazon.com/dp/B00HHGRBBQ

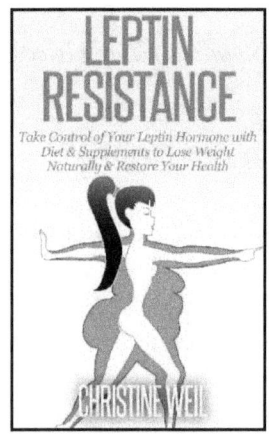

http://www.amazon.com/dp/B00J8UNBWW

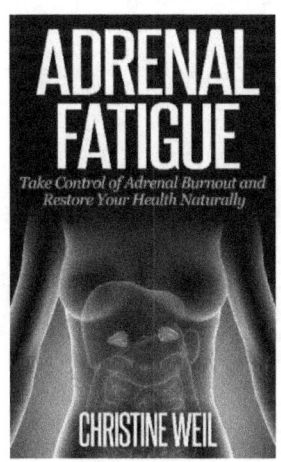

http://www.amazon.com/dp/B00J8SHS6E

References:

*Recipes from *The Naturally Clean Home* by Karyn Siegel-Maier.

Grow Your own Drugs by James Wong

Guide to Healing Herbs, Volume 2 Published by Mother Earth News

*www.herbcompanion.com

*Medline Plus. "Eucalyptus: MedlinePlus Supplements ." 2012. www.nlm.nih.gov/ medlineplus/ druginfo/ natural/ 700. Html

*Bramble, Arthur (2014-01-07). Herbal Remedies Bible: Life Saving And Healing Herbs For All Ailments : Easy Herbal Remedies For Over 100 Ailments (p. 106).